TRICK YOURSELF INTO LOSING WEIGHT

A Psychiatrist's Guide to Dieting

By **Robert Elias, M.D.**
Edited By **Stephen Elias**

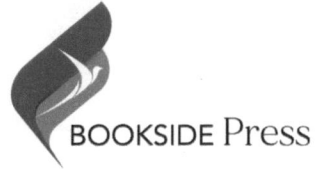

BOOKSIDE Press

Copyright © 2024 by Robert Elias, M.D.

ISBN: 978-1-77883-429-5 (Paperback)

978-1-77883-430-1 (E-book)

All rights reserved. No part of this publication may be reproduced, distributed, or transmitted in any form or by any means, including photocopying, recording, or other electronic or mechanical methods, without the prior written permission of the publisher, except in the case brief quotations embodied in critical reviews and other noncommercial uses permitted by copyright law.

The views expressed in this book are solely those of the author and do not necessarily reflect the views of the publisher, and the publisher hereby disclaims any responsibility for them.

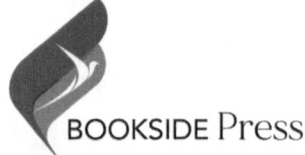

BookSide Press
877-741-8091
www.booksidepress.com
orders@booksidepress.com

To Lois

Contents

Introduction vii
Chapter 1	Should you return this book?.	1
Chapter 2	Why lose weight	3
Chapter 3	How food interacts with the body	9
Chapter 4	Why diets don't work.	.12
Chapter 5	The American eating disease	.17
Chapter 6	Denial is not a river in Egypt.	.22
Chapter 7	Getting started	.25
Chapter 8	Calories count and the air does not contain them . . .	.36
Chapter 9	No second helpings.	.40
Chapter 10	Dealing with addictive foods	.43
Chapter 11	Eating out	.45
Chapter 12	Tricks and triggers	.53
Chapter 13	First step-stabilizing your weight	.56
Chapter 14	Resting or turning eating efforts into eating habits . .	.60
Chapter 15	Making a plan to lose weight.	.61
Chapter 16	Resting after a weight loss	.65
Chapter 17	Holiday eating	.66
Chapter 18	Quitting smoking	.68
Chapter 19	Traveling	.69

Introduction

My background is in Medicine and Psychiatry. I have been practicing psychiatry for the past 37 years, working with people to change faulty habits in living. It occurred to me that our current problem with failed weight control in this country might be approached in a similar manner, as faulty habits in eating.

The psychotherapeutic process is one that takes a long time. The psyche tends to resist change. One must be very patient with people who are attempting to grow psychologically. There are steps forward and back. Progress occurs and then seems to recede. Many psychological problems do not respond to advice or short-term methods. We tend to think of needing years rather than months for improvement to occur. One must be very attentive to signs of resistance and they need to be examined and talked about before real change can occur.

In dieting, also, we need to address the resistance to change. Although important, it is not enough to simply figure out how many calories to cut or what foods not to eat. Attention needs to be paid to the psychology of "purposeful eating" and the resistance to change in our eating habits.

It seems clear by now that we don't know what to do about our weight problem in this country, except of course to write books about it. Amazon.com has 15,475 responses to the book search for "diet". In spite of all these books, however, we continue to gain weight. In fact we have begun to realize that obesity in the United States is one of our very worst health problems.

I don't simply wish to make the list of diet books. That would be a waste of money and good paper. I present a somewhat different slant on the process of dealing with our weight problems. This book focuses on our resistance to weight loss, and how to deal with it, not only the nuts and bolts of dieting. I think that this is important because most people who try to lose weight fail. When one thinks about it, this is somewhat surprising. We are very successful at combating many of our health problems. Even the dreaded cancer is giving way to the constant onslaught from science and technology. Failed organs can be replaced; livers, kidneys, hearts, hips, and knees. But somehow obesity remains a devilishly difficult problem.

The words diet and dieting will be used in this book and would seem to be a contradiction as the theme of this book is to lose weight without dieting. The words are used simply for lack of any better ones to express generally what we are trying to do.

This book, as it is currently arranged, presents background and scientific material first and the nuts and bolts of how to lose weight later. If you desire to get right to the heart of the matter, you may wish to skip the early chapters and start with Chapter 7 Getting Started.

If you are browsing in a bookstore right now, you may want to read Chapter 1, "Should you return this book", before you buy it.

1

Should you return this book?

There have been lots of books written about diets. High Protein, Low Protein, High Fat, Low Fat, High Carbohydrate, Low Carbohydrate, Grapefruit, etc. etc. Probably all of them work for a while but only for a while. Diets in general don't work in the long run and money spent for books about them usually are a waste. I don't want to contribute to this wastage so before you begin this book look over the following questions to get some idea of what you're getting yourself into.

- Many diet books promise quick results. This one will not. If you're looking for the six-week method to lose 100 pounds then this is not the book for you. On the other hand, even if progress is slow, the approach I advocate will not be uncomfortable, and the weight you lose will stay off.

- Examining your eating-out habits will be crucial to your progress. Are you willing to make some changes in your eating-out patterns and perhaps curtail some of the huge portions that you receive?

- Rather than devising a diet that you can let go of once you achieve your goal, my approach involves a life-long change. Each step must be carefully considered. Are you up for this?

- My approach requires that you more or less keep track of what you eat and examine the dietary information in all your meals. Then you will need to make rules for yourself with respect to what you eat. Perhaps "limits" is a better word. With respect to food we are all children. We want what we want. As children our parents set limits for us. "Only one scoop of ice-cream and then to bed". As adults we wouldn't put up with this. So we have to make our own limits and learn to live by them. This will be somewhat difficult at first. But once you achieve a bit of success I think you will find the process very rewarding and easier as you go along.

2

Why lose weight

I presume that you bought this book because you're overweight and want to do something about it. Even so it probably won't hurt to go over some reasons for shedding some pounds.

By far the most important reason for losing weight is your health. Diabetes, Heart disease, Arthritis, and High Blood Pressure, are just a few of the common consequences of being overweight. These are all serious conditions and can impact your life in unimaginably negative ways—shortening it for example. In addition, you may be concerned about your appearance, or the ability to fit into an airplane seat. Or you may be limiting your ability to engage in various physical activities due to the difficulty in lugging around those extra pounds. It may be that your doctor has told you that you need to lose weight in order to help reduce your blood pressure or a high fasting blood sugar level, which could mean diabetes if left untreated.

Whether you are obese or just "overweight" is a somewhat difficult question. The United States Department of Health and Human Resources publishes tables of "desirable" weights related only to one's height for men and women together. For example the desirable weight for a person in the 1996 tables who is 5 feet 8 inches tall is between

125 and 164 pounds. This does not distinguish between any of many personal physical characteristics including gender, bone and muscle sizes. Indeed, it is hard to see how these numbers could be very helpful in making a decision about whether you should lose weight and if so, how much.

The other currently popular means of determining overweightness is by calculating the body mass index or BMI. This is also a method of relating your weight to your height without taking into consideration the difference in weight between a heavily and lightly muscled individual, male or female, and so on. So, I also hesitate to get into this area of conflict. Rather, I suggest you consult your family doctor or a dietician for a personal assessment of only you, in terms of whether or not you need to lose weight. That being said I will go ahead and define obesity according to what in my opinion are flawed standards so that there are some numbers to compare yourself against—taking into account your particular body type.

The Body Mass Index is calculated by taking your weight in Kilograms and dividing it by your height in meters squared. To get your weight in Kilos divide your weight in pounds by 2.2. To get your height in meters divide your height in inches by 39.

Let's take an example:

Your weight is 200 pounds. Your height is five foot eight inches or 68 inches (5x12+8). Your weight in Kilos is 200 divided by 2.2 equals 90.90. Your height in meters is 68 divided by 39 equals 1.74. To square it you multiply it by itself: 1.74x1.74 equals 3.034. Next you divide 90.90 by 3.034 equals 30 (rounded off from 29.96). This is your Body Mass Index. The following ranges are arbitrarily chosen and given names such as normal, overweight, obese and so on. Also see table 1.

18.5-24.9 Normal
25-29.9 Overweight
30-and above, Obese

Table 1

BODY MASS INDEX

| | 19 | 20 | 21 | 22 | 23 | 24 | 25 | 26 | 27 | 28 | 29 | 30 | 31 | 32 | 33 | 34 | 35 |

Height (Inches)   Body weight (pounds)

Height	19	20	21	22	23	24	25	26	27	28	29	30	31	32	33	34	35
58	91	96	100	105	110	115	119	124	129	134	138	143	148	153	158	162	167
59	94	99	104	109	114	119	124	128	133	138	143	148	153	158	163	168	173
60	97	102	107	112	118	123	128	133	138	143	148	153	158	163	168	174	179
61	100	106	111	116	122	127	132	137	143	148	153	158	164	169	174	180	185
62	104	109	115	120	126	131	136	142	147	153	158	164	169	175	180	186	191
63	107	113	118	124	130	135	141	146	152	158	163	169	175	180	186	191	197
64	110	116	122	128	134	140	145	151	157	163	169	174	180	186	192	197	204
65	114	120	126	132	138	144	150	156	162	168	174	180	186	192	198	204	210
66	118	124	130	136	142	148	155	161	167	173	179	186	192	198	204	210	216
67	121	127	134	140	146	153	159	166	172	178	185	191	198	204	211	217	223
68	125	131	138	144	151	158	164	171	177	184	190	197	203	210	216	223	230
69	128	135	142	149	155	162	169	176	182	189	196	203	209	216	223	230	236
70	132	139	146	153	160	167	174	181	188	195	202	209	216	222	229	236	243
71	136	143	150	157	165	172	179	186	193	200	208	215	222	229	236	243	250
72	140	147	154	162	169	177	184	191	199	206	213	221	228	235	242	250	258
73	144	151	159	166	174	182	189	197	204	212	219	227	235	242	250	257	265
74	148	155	163	171	179	186	194	202	210	218	225	233	241	249	256	264	272
75	152	160	168	176	184	192	200	208	216	224	232	240	248	256	264	272	279
76	156	164	172	180	189	197	205	213	221	230	238	246	254	263	271	279	287

To use this table, find your height in the left-hand column. Move across to your weight. The number at the top is your body mass index. Normal is defined as 19-25. Overweight is defined as 25-30. Obese is defined as over 30.

There is overwhelming evidence that obesity is a marked health risk. According to the 2002 edition of "Current Medical Diagnosis and Treatment" published by McGraw Hill those that are 30 percent overweight have an increased mortality rate of 30 percent. Those at 50 percent overweight increase their mortality rate by 100 percent, and at 100 percent have a 1,000 percent increase in mortality rate. For example, suppose you determine with your doctor that your desirable weight is 150 pounds and you actually weigh 195 pounds. You are 30 percent overweight. If you weigh 225 pounds you are 50 percent overweight. If you weigh 300 pounds you are 100 percent overweight.

What are Mortality Rates?

Mortality rates are statistical values gathered for any particular grouping usually by age and gender. In this case a statistical value is a number that tells you how many people will die each year for any reason including illnesses, accidents, etc. It doesn't tell you what you will die from, just that you will die. This is expressed as a percentage, or the number of people who died out of 100. 3 percent would be 3 out of 100. To say that you have an *increased* mortality rate of 30 percent and let's say for your age and gender the average mortality rate is 3 percent (3 people die for every 100 that year), 30 percent of 3 is about 1, so 4 people out of 100 will die that year. It doesn't mean that *you* will, but in a large group of people 30 percent overweight it will work out that on average 4 people out of 100 in your age and gender range will die that year instead of 3 in a population of normal weight individuals.

It always strikes me that the manner in which numbers are expressed has a great deal to do with their emotional impact. In the above "30 percent more die" is scarier than "your chances of dying from this go from 3 to 4 out of 100". As the percentages go up it gets scarier, however. The individual who is 50 percent overweight increased his or her being in the group of people who die that year from 3 out of 100 to 6 out of 100. The person who is 100 percent overweight increased his or her being in the group dying that year from 3 out of 100 to 30 out of 100.

Diabetes and Obesity

According to recent statistics sixteen million Americans are diabetic and 800,000 more become diabetic every year. Harvard researchers have determined that between 50 and 75 percent of new cases of diabetes result from people being overweight. Diabetes has been shown conclusively to be a direct cause of heart disease, stroke, kidney failure, blindness, and the loss of limbs by amputation. Unfortunately, by the time the diagnosis is made the damage is often done. Many studies have shown that even a modest degree of weight loss can prevent the onset of diabetes. In one study a weight loss of only ten pounds reduced the incidence of diabetes in overweight people by 30 percent.

Hypertension and Obesity

Hypertension (high blood pressure) sometimes is called "the silent killer" because often you can't tell you have it until the damage is done. Hypertension is associated with a higher degree of heart disease, kidney disease, and stroke and dementia (such as Alzheimer's disease). Hypertension can often quite effectively be treated with weight loss alone. Joe, a patient of mine, is muscular and athletic. He is about 5 feet 8 inches tall and weighs about 215-220 pounds. His blood pressure runs high enough to require treatment with 2 antihypertensives (medications that reduce blood pressure). He decided to lose weight. He was able to get his weight down (by going on a strict diet) to 195 pounds. His blood pressure returned to normal. Unfortunately he was unable to keep the weight off due to the fact that he lost weight by strict dieting rather than changing his eating habits. You guessed it. His hypertension returned.

Obesity and Other Disorders

Another disorder that occurs in greater frequency in obese people is degenerative joint disease or Osteoarthritis. The extra weight carried on the cartilage in the weight bearing joints tends to wear out faster leading to immobility and chronic pain in those joints. Colorectal cancer, prostate cancer, uterine cancer, breast and ovarian cancers, gallstones, and reflux esophagitis are other disorders that occur in greater frequency in obese individuals. In addition surgical and obstetric risks are greater.

3

How food interacts with the body

There are three basic types of food; proteins, carbohydrates, and fats. The way in which food is transformed so that it can be used by the body is called the metabolism. The basal metabolism is the amount of calories burned at rest.

Proteins are what we use to build and maintain the physical plant of our bodies. They are constructed from chemicals called amino acids. We get most of our amino acids from eating proteins and breaking them down into their constituent amino acids. The amino acids that we can only get from eating proteins are called essential amino acids. Non-essential amino acids can be made by the body. Some sources of proteins contain all the essential amino acids and some don't. You must have all the essential amino acids in order to live. The most complete source for essential amino acids is meat. Cuisines that do not include meat, have, over the eons, combined other sources of proteins in combinations so that all the essential amino acids are included. The rice, beans, and corn cuisine of Mexico is a good example of this.

Carbohydrates are foods that we get from vegetables and grains. Green vegetables, starchy vegetables such as potatoes and rice, and grains such as wheat are all sources of carbohydrates. Carbohydrates are composed of various combinations of sugars, which the body breaks down into a chemical called glucose. Glucose is then broken down even further by various chemical processes to yield packets of energy. The body needs these to do all it's tasks such as contracting muscles (including the heart and intestines), operating the big computer upstairs (the brain), digesting food, making blood cells, repairing the body when it is damaged, and so on.

Carbohydrates are necessary for life. This is because the various chemical processes mentioned above will not work without glucose. Without glucose the body will not have any of the packets of energy to run all its machinery. The liver and muscles store some extra carbohydrate in the form of a molecule called glycogen. This will last a day or two if no carbohydrates are taken in. Then the body starts breaking down muscles tissue in order to free up some extra amino acids in order to manufacture some glucose. This is important to understand because some of the means of dieting being sold to Americans today involve depriving the body of glucose. Low carbohydrate diets are discussed further in Chapter #4 why diets don't work.

Fats are basically a means by which the body stores excess food. It's essential to the survival of any species that has an intermittent food supply. The Human species hasn't always had a hamburger stand on the corner or a neighborhood market teeming with any food that you might desire. During much of our history food was available intermittently. After a good hunt, or a very successful food gather, people ate as much as they could. The excess was deposited in the body as fat. Then, during those lean times when game was not available or there was nothing to gather, the body used the excess fat to run all the machinery until the next source of food was available. Fat is a very efficient means of energy storage. Each gram of fat yields 9 calories of energy. Each gram of protein and carbohydrate yields only 4 calories. Fats are also necessary for life even in a society, which has a regular supply of food.

Many vitamins are fat-soluble and depend upon the presence of fats in the body for availability. In addition certain fatty acids are nec- essary for the production of vital bodily chemicals.

4

Why diets don't work

The fundamental problem with attempting to lose weight is that your body will fight you every step of the way. There are numerous hormonal and neurological mechanisms designed to maintain body weight. These systems are critical to all living things, as it is vital that all organisms have a means of knowing when they need more food and stimulating them to do something about it. Some of these systems are known and many aren't.

New discoveries about hunger

Hunger is understood to originate in a particular area of the brain known as the hypothalamus. The hypothalamus is stimulated by messages from other areas of the brain and from reduced levels of nutrients in the blood such as glucose. A recent discovery has shown that a hormone originating in the stomach and small intestine called ghrelin also stimulates the hypothalamus—producing the sensation of hunger. The levels of ghrelin in the blood vary throughout the day and are highest right before meals. In a small study involving 13 people, the researchers discovered that after losing about 17 percent of their body weight, these folks had significantly higher level of ghrelin throughout the day. The more weight an individual had lost, the bigger the post-diet increase in ghrelin levels. This interesting discovery offers proof of at least one system whose aim is to restore lost body weight. It should be noted that it doesn't matter how much you weigh for this system to take effect. The body doesn't appreciate normal weight charts and the like. It just wants that weight back.

Diets often work in the short run but not in the long run because there is too much weight lost in a short period and there is no plan for keeping the weight off. Many diets involve a marked change in eating habits and change in food over a short period of time, and then—almost inevitably—a return to the old eating habits. A good example of this is the low carbohydrate, high fat and protein diet. It used to be called the drinking man's diet because alcohol is the result of carbohydrates being broken down by the processes involved in creating the alcoholic beverage and doesn't count in adding up the amount of carbohydrate you ate that day. The trouble with this diet is that you are basically starving yourself by not eating enough carbohydrates to run your metabolism. A certain minimum amount of carbohydrate is required in order for your metabolism to work (in other words you can't live without them). These diets are based on you eating less than this minimum amount. The body then attempts to compensate by breaking down fats and proteins.

The way you tell if you are doing a low-carbohydrate diet right is to measure the ketones (the chemicals that result from breaking down fats) in your urine. They tend to be acidic and in sufficient amounts produce an acidic condition in the blood called ketoacidosis. There are little strips of paper that turn purple in the presence of ketones. Ketonuria (ketones measured in the urine) is one of the signs of diabetic ketoacidosis (a severe potentially fatal result of uncontrolled diabetes). This weight loss can be dramatic but as soon as you stop and go back to your prior eating habits, the weight comes right back. And you certainly will go back to your old eating habits. No one could stay on one of these diets for very long as they make you feel tired and ill. Worse, you have probably lowered your metabolic rate and so will put on even more weight than you lost. One of the ways the body reacts to weight loss is to lower the basal metabolic rate (the amount of energy used at rest) in order to try and preserve as much body mass as possible. In olden times, during times of food shortage, this was an adaptation that prolonged the lives and passed on the genes of those who could do it.

Proponents of the Atkins diet, a diet of high fat and protein, and low complex carbohydrates, will argue that ketones are natures response to an intermittent food supply and a fine source of energy for the body during times of food shortage. This is undoubtedly true and we are certainly fortunate to have such a back up system. It begs the question, however, that in the presence of adequate food, people will be unlikely to undergo the unpleasantness of ketosis (ketones in the blood, see above). And again, as I keep harping, there is no plan for what happens after you lose the weight you want and return to normal eating. The Adkins diet has not been well accepted by the medical establishment. Lately however, there has been a resurgence of interest. This is due to increasing evidence that link the epidemic of obesity to the high carbohydrate-low fat diets in vogue over the past 20 to 30 years. Grants have recently been provided to study the benefits and drawbacks of the Adkins diet.

How about the grapefruit diet. People lose weight like crazy. But when you're through, what then. Keep eating nothing but grapefruit? I don't think so. Back to Pizza and Hamburgers.

There are many diets on the market that involve buying certain products that you eat instead of your regular food. I guess they work in the short term; at least the people who sell them say so. But what about later when you stop because you're tired of milk shakes three times per day and it's time to go back to normal food? You resume your prior eating habits and the owner of the so-called diet sends his kid off to an expensive eastern university.

There are appetite suppressant medications that generally involve stimulants. They work by tricking the body into thinking that it is not hungry. They do this by increasing serotonin or catecholamine, two brain chemicals that affect mood and appetite. The appetite depressant effect tends to wear off after a few weeks. It is not recommended that these medications be taken indefinitely due to potentially hazardous side effects. Some have recently been taken off the market because of serious health risks, which may include valvular heart disease.

Fat absorption inhibitors work by preventing your body from breaking down and absorbing fat eaten with your meals. These are prescription medications that have been approved for longer-term use in significantly obese people. The safety and effectiveness have not been approved for use longer than one year. They have been shown to be moderately effective but not for periods longer than 6 months.

Everyone knows that there's more than one way to skin a cat. That goes for weight loss too. Mention should be made of group-supported diets such as weight watchers or overeaters anonymous. These groups have been very helpful to many people seeking to lose weight. I would certainly encourage anyone so inclined to enter one of these organizations. Of course not everyone is a joiner and not everyone would feel comfortable talking about his or her weight problem in front of strangers. But for those who would, this would be an effective adjunct to what I am proposing here. The main benefit here in my opinion is the group support. One downside is that some of them have products for you to buy. This should always be suspect because you must consider what's going to happen when you no longer wish to purchase these products—which can be rather expensive. I think that any sudden change in eating habits followed by a return to your regular eating habits is doomed to fail and may in fact lead in the end to a rise in weight.

5

The American eating disease

I recently received the following email, which is circulating around cyberspace

"The Japanese eat very little fat and suffer fewer heart attacks than the British or Americans"
"On the other hand, the French eat a lot of fat and also suffer fewer heart attacks than the British or Americans."
"The Chinese drink very little red wine and suffer fewer heart attacks than the British or Americans."
"The Italians drink excessive amounts of red wine and also suffer fewer heart attacks than the British or Americans."
"Conclusion: Eat and drink what you like. It's speaking English that kills you."

If Osama Bin Laden were really as smart as everyone thinks he is he would have spent his millions on buying several of the popular fast-food franchises rather than on terrorist attacks and wait for us all to eat ourselves to death. In the United States, obesity is implicated in the deaths of 300,000 people annually from heart disease, stroke, diabetes, and cancer. The truth is, obesity is an American Eating Disease.

The statistics are staggering. Nearly 65% of adults and 15 % of children ages 6-19 in the American population are overweight and about 33% of the population are considered to be Obese. Obesity is discussed in more detail in chapter 2. Adult onset diabetes, a consequence of obesity, is a raging epidemic. See chapter 2 for more on diabetes. This year (2004) 60,000 Americans who are morbidly obese (100 pounds or more overweight) will have major surgery to seal off most of their stomachs and shorten their intestines to lose weight.

Our lifestyle may be partly to blame. The industrial revolution created machines that have virtually replaced all human labor. Almost all work is sedentary. Automobiles take us from place to place with the caloric expenditure equivalent to sitting and watching TV.

The movement of women out of the home and into the workplace during the latter half of the 20th century has lead to a marked change in our eating habits. There is little energy left over to cook. The family meal has gone by the wayside. 40 percent of all food is eaten out. The fast food industry has supplied the nation with cheap, very tasty meals that we obtain on the run. Perhaps the emotional nourishment we received from family contact at mealtime has been replaced to a certain degree with more food. Competition between these large chain restaurants has resulted in ever-larger meals and tempting television ads that tempt us to eat more than we need. Advertising for food chains is hard to resist. The ads make those meals so appetizing that one can hardly finish the TV program without leaving to go get that burger with three meat patties or lobster and shrimp with cheese bread. See chapter #14 for more on eating out and how to deal with the large portions of food served.

With the advent of modern electronics, children are increasingly entertained by video games and television programs, which are markedly sedentary activities. This is in marked contrast to prior generations of children who played outdoors and tended to move around more.

The more food you eat, the more money is made by the U.S. food industry. Never forget this. It pervades every eating activity in which we partake—even something as simple as buying ground beef or turkey. I noticed during the past few years that when I went to my local large chain supermarket to shop for the ingredients for my spaghetti sauce, the packets of ground beef had grown from one pound to one and one quarter pounds. Of course I could push the ringer and the butcher would have made me a one-pound packet. But since I was in a rush, as we all are in this country, I didn't bother. So in my spaghetti sauce recipe there was an extra 25% of ground beef. Last week the packets suddenly contained 1.35 pounds. I dug around under all the packets and at the very bottom found one with 1.13 pounds—but never just a pound.

The U.S. Dept. of Agriculture has data showing that 3,800 calories worth of food per person is produced in the U.S. every day. This is about twice what we need. Their data related to dietary intake shows a 236-calorie per person per day increase between 1987 and 1995. That translates into a 24-pound weight gain per person every year. Much of the increase comes from prepared food that is enriched with sugar and fat. They found that added sugar is found in such foods as pizza, bread, hot dogs, soup, crackers, spaghetti sauce, lunchmeat, canned vegetables, fruit drinks, flavored yogurt, ketchup, salad dressing, and mayonnaise.

About ten percent of all calories ingested in this country come from soda pop. This is not surprising to anyone who frequents a market as about ten percent of the shelf space is taken up by sodas. We have allowed ourselves to be hoodwinked into substituting soda pop for water. There is something very subtle about this that undermines reasonable eating habits. If you order a soda at a restaurant or buy one at the store you almost certainly finish it. You drink all of it because it tastes good—not because you need more fluid at that particular time. Sadly, soda pop is being sold in our public schools. The schools have contractual arrangements with the soda pop companies and receive a portion of the income. They have come to depend on this income to run part of the their school programs. The average teenager drinks about three sodas per day. The city of Los Angeles school district, attempting to combat the increasing obesity epidemic, is considering banning the sale of soft drinks on its 677 campuses. The profits from these sales average $39,000 per high school and $14,000 per middle school.

Never Forget the Bottom Line

The most important figure in this country is the bottom line. Don't expect much help from the government with this problem. A growing economy (and waistline) however, is just fine with all concerned. If Safeway, for example, can sell more beef, then they can buy more beef from the wholesaler. The wholesaler can pay more to the rancher who can pay more for the feed and the farm machinery. And they all can then pay more taxes. You can then pay more to the healthcare industry, not only for medical treatment but also for research into cures for the many diseases that result from obesity. In my humble opinion, a "war on food" should be substituted for the "war on drugs".

Apparently to accommodate the physical growth of the American population, the clothing industry is doing something very strange. It's called "vanity sizing". They are actually changing the sizes of women's clothing. By that I mean that if you're a size 14 you are probably buying size 12 and so on. I guess if you're a gal and you go into an expensive boutique and can't struggle into your usual size you're not going to buy the item. So in some back room a bunch of clever business persons figured out what to do. Just lower the numbers. And they did. I'm not sure why they haven't for men. I would love to believe that my waist size is the same as when I was in junior high school. It's just not fair. The point I'm trying to make here is that we wish to be in denial about our weight, and far be it for any industry whether it is food or clothing to get in the way of our denial.

6

Denial is not a river in Egypt

Psychological defense mechanisms discovered by Sigmund Freud serve us in many ways. They also disserve us in many ways. Defense mechanisms serve to protect us from anxiety. For example the mechanism of repression keeps us from experiencing and acting on most of the unpleasant and antisocial impulses present in the unconscious. For example, many violent and sexual impulses that are present in early life must be pushed down (repressed) in order to allow us to function in our families and in society.

Rationalization is another common defense in which we make reasons for doing or not doing things that might make us anxious if we were to understand the full import of what we were doing. For example, we might wish to spend a lot of money on the purchase of a new car. The old car does not need to really be replaced and the new car costs much more than we can really afford. So we make up compelling reasons to go ahead. A frequent reason that you give yourself is that you don't want to put money into the old car. Often what is being defended against is guilt about impulsively spending money on oneself and especially when you can't afford it and the rest of the family is going to be deprived of something more essential than a new car. The reasons that we give ourselves are called rationalization. This is a particularly effective defense mechanism as any wife who tries to talk her husband out of buying a new shiny sports car can attest to. Of course the smart wife will simply say, "No, you can't do that". But if you try to engage the defense mechanism by arguing with it you don't get very far.

Denial is another primitive defense mechanism that is somewhat akin to sticking your head in the sand. I think we see it frequently in dealing with health risks and the many dangers lurking in our world. Denial does what the word implies, that is, one denies the fact, feeling, of whatever one doesn't want to acknowledge. For example people who engage in unprotected sex in the midst of a very serious HIV epidemic with risk to their lives are saying in effect "I deny that this can happen to me". When I was a medical student in San Francisco I once was assigned a liver failure case on one of the wards at San Francisco General Hospital. The man had a lengthy history of alcoholism. As I approached his bed the aroma of alcoholic spirits wafted around me. I introduced myself and began the interview. After inquiring into his general health and living situation, I finally got around to asking him how much he had been drinking lately. "Lately?" he slurringly asked. "I haven't had a drink in months". That was classic denial.

These defense mechanisms also are quite necessary for dealing with some of the unpleasant realities that we, as conscious human beings, know to be true. We know we're going to die, sometime, but hopefully we don't go about our daily lives thinking about it. Instead we tend to think, "it won't happen to me" (denial) or "if I eat right and get a lot of exercise, I'll prevent death from happening to me for the foreseeable future" (rationalization). Another example. I live in a small California city. We are not prone to the numbers of homicides that occur in the bigger cities. So, I don't think about it much. One morning the daily newspaper reported a robbery murder in my city. I remember looking for the location within the city and thinking to myself with relief that it wasn't in my section of the city and therefore not a threat to my family or I. A few months later the same thing happened but this time in my section. So I searched for the street and felt relief that it wasn't my street.

So, you may be thinking, what does all this have to do with eating? In spite of overwhelming evidence that is available to everyone that obesity is a substantial health threat and life-shortening problem, few obese people go around thinking about how they are taking years off their lives. They don't think about the fact that the two thousand calorie meal they just consumed is going to make it worse, or that their weight has been getting worse for years and the situation is pretty much hopeless—unless drastic changes in their eating behavior are made. Instead it goes something like this: "I know that I'm a little heavy but it's a temporary problem and next year I'm going to do something about it", or "sure I overdid it at dinner last night but I'll make up for it tomorrow by eating less", or "I may be a bit heavy but so was my father (mother) and he (she) lived to be eighty five". Of course now we have modern medicine to help us rationalize our eating behavior. Now we can say "sure I'm overweight but my cholesterol is normal so I don't have to worry". You get the idea.

In a Harvard University survey released in May 2002, more than half of those surveyed said they were overweight. But 78 percent of those overweight people did not think their weight was a problem. Though a vast majority regarded cancer, AIDS, and heart disease as serious health problems, only a third of those surveyed thought obesity was.

Now take a few moments to think about how you, personally, defend against the anxiety associated with your particular eating and weight problem and thus keep yourself from doing anything about it.

7

Getting started

The core idea of this book

By making small adjustments in calorie intake over a long period of time, you will painlessly (without gnawing feelings of hunger) eat less and therefore weigh less. This will be a regimen of foods chosen by you. There will be no instructions in this book to eat this or don't eat that. A diet based on that sort of advice is doomed to fail. I will make suggestions about what foods are full of fat and it might help to eat a little less of them. Also I can't promise not to get on you about eating more vegetables, as you will see.

Gathering some Source Materials

First you'll need a book of food values. I use Corinne T. Netzer's "The Complete Book of Food Counts". This will tell you how many grams of protein, fat, carbohydrates, and calories are in just about anything you eat, including prepared and frozen foods. It will be important to learn that, unit for unit, fat contains more than twice the calories of protein or carbohydrate. What makes it harder from a dieting standpoint is that fats, along with sugar, are what give our food flavor. Anything that tastes really good does so because of the fat and sugar it contains. In time it will become important to adjust the fat content of your food so that it tastes good, but not too good, if you know what I mean. If you try and get rid of all the fat in your diet, you won't like your food much and you won't like your diet much.

"Restaurant Confidential" by Jacobson and Hurley will give you the caloric, fat and sodium content of restaurant food including all of the big chains. This book is especially helpful if you eat out frequently. This subject will be discussed in more detail in chapter 11.

Understanding measurements

To understand the food you are eating, it will help to understand the words used on the packages when disclosing measurement information about their contents. Measures of food are often expressed in the metric system. Food weights on packages are usually expressed in grams. There are one thousand grams in a Kilogram. There are about 30 grams in an ounce. There are 16 ounces in a pound. A kilogram weighs 2.2 pounds. Please take the time to understand these numbers so that you'll be able to understand the Nutrition Facts you encounter in the Supermarket.

Reading the Package

All packaged foods have "Nutrition Facts" somewhere on the package. On the first line is serving size. For example the cracker box I'm looking at right now says the serving size is five crackers. Everything else on the label is related to the serving size. The calories (80) are per serving size (5 crackers). The calories from fat are 30 per serving size or 5 crackers. The Total Fat (3.5 g-grams) is per serving size or 5 crackers. The fat is broken down into saturated, polyunsaturated, and monounsaturated. If you subtract these last three fats from the total fat you'll get the transfat. Transfat is made artificially by putting hydrogen atoms on fat that is liquid at room temperature such as cooking oil. This is called hydrogenation and causes the oil to become solid at room temperature. This is increasingly thought to be a factor in heart disease. Most likely, the transfat values will be listed in the "nutritional facts" box in the near future. There also is information regarding Cholesterol, Sodium, Total Carbohydrate, Dietary fiber, sugars, and Protein. Some vitamins, Calcium, and Iron content are listed. Lastly are values for recommended daily allowances for Total fat, Saturated fat, Cholesterol, Sodium, Total Carbohydrate, and Dietary fiber.

Buy a calculator

Now is the time to buy a calculator if you don't already have one. The first step is to write down in a diary what you typically eat, and then figure out how many calories are involved. While you're at it, you can figure out what the percentages of fat, especially saturated fat, are in your diet.

Pay close attention to fat

Knowing about the fat content of your food is important because, as mentioned, fat contains at least twice the calories as does carbohydrate or protein; 9 calories per gram to 4 calories per gram. Therefore by substituting a small amount of carbohydrate or protein for an equivalent amount of fat one can easily cut out some calories without affecting the bulk or size of your portions.

Another important reason for coming to terms with information regarding fat is that the current conventional wisdom regarding fat intake is that it should not exceed 35% of your calories. (By the way, this figure was just increased from 30% by the U.S.D.A). These are labeled as "fat calories" on the package. I think that there is some confusion between the amount of fat in a given dish and the amount of fat that is allowed in a day. For example, just because some item has, say, 80 percent fat calories doesn't mean that you can't have it. It's the percent of your total daily caloric intake that fat calories represent that is significant.

Of course as time goes on and you get into this process, you will be interested in those highly fatty foods because they offer a greater potential for reducing calories in your diet than do carbohydrates and protein. The 35 percent mark is hard to reach, but certainly not impossible. I certainly would not suggest trying to go below 35%. This will take the flavor out of your food as well as making you get hungry sooner. Food that "sticks to your ribs" does so in large part because of the fat (and protein) it contains.

I think I need to put a disclaimer in here about the health risks of fat. This is a rather confusing subject. The conventional wisdom is, of course, that fat is bad. This conventional wisdom has been with us for about 25-30 years. There is some evidence, however, to suggest that our current obesity epidemic may be related more to our obsession with cutting fat out of our diets than to the fat itself. The sudden jump in overweight percentages in this country nearly coincides with the medical establishment's edict regarding the evils of fat. Eating large amounts of carbohydrates (instead of fats) may result in a larger intake of calories overall. Attention is now being directed toward carbohydrates that are easily broken down into glucose such as foods made with white flour, pasta, potatoes and other starches. There is even a new terminology for this called the Glycemic Index.

Food with a high Glycemic index is food that gets a lot of glucose into your blood very fast—and which therefore stimulates the release of large amounts of insulin. This increased insulin, so the theory goes, causes glucose to go into the cells faster leading us to be hungry sooner and consume more food. Interestingly, the percent of recommended fat in your diet that for many years has been 30 percent (as described above) has recently been upgraded to 35 percent by the U.S.D.A. They are also starting to tinker with those little food pyramids that no one I know pays attention to.

There is also the problem of the bad cholesterol (low-density lipoprotein) and the good cholesterol (high-density lipoprotein). If you cut out all that wonderfully good tasting saturated fat from your diet you may reduce your bad cholesterol but you may also reduce your good cholesterol.

While these issues are being studied and debated, I don't think you would be remiss if you took the ancient Greek attitude of "moderation in all things" and apply that to your eating habits.

Understanding calories or Calories 101

It is probably clear to you now that in order to get a hold of your weight problem you will need to become familiar with calories—what they are and how managing them will help you lose weight. Calories are units of energy that we get from the food that we eat. Depending on our weight, level of physical activity, basal metabolism, and other factors we will need a certain number of calories per day to maintain our weight. If we eat more than this amount of calories we will gain weight and if we eat less we will lose weight. We need between 12 and 15 calories per pound to maintain our weight depending upon our level of physical activity. If we can cut the number of calories needed to maintain a pound of body weight (12-15) then we will lose it over time.

Each pound of body mass is equivalent to 3500 calories. So, if we can eat 3500 calories less than we need to maintain our weight, we will lose a pound. How fast or slow we will lose weight depends on how many fewer calories we eat each day than what we need. Slow is probably better in the long run because our bodies won't fight as hard to keep the weight on. Please see chapter 8 for more information on calories and how this 3500 calorie figure fits into the larger strategy of losing weight.

Exercise can help

I guess I should say something about exercise. Everyone else does. The trouble with connecting exercise to the problem of weight control is that it's the same problem as crash dieting. It's great but will you keep doing it? Most people who join a gym and exercise like crazy for a while usually don't keep it up. I would suggest instead finding something that you really enjoy and do that (because it's healthful and fun) but don't expect it to have much impact on your weight problem, although it may help some. I was amazed to learn that a marathon runner only loses one pound of true body weight (what's left after the salt and fluids are put back) during a marathon. It takes a reduction of 3500 calories below what you need to maintain your weight to lose one pound. If you divide 3500 by 26 (miles) you get about 135 calories lost per mile run. 135 calories are contained in a bowl of soup, a little more than a piece of bread, a piece of fruit, one drink, etc. That's a lot of work for very few calories unless it's something you really love to do anyway. Nevertheless, a short pleasant walk several times a week may burn some extra calories and may also benefit your cardiovascular system.

Exercise and Modern Living

Someone did a study a few years ago about how many calories it takes to do all those little things we no longer do because of technology. For example how many calories do you use to get up and change the channel on the TV rather than use the remote? I think it might have been four calories. In any event it added up over a whole day to quite a few. There is a very funny movie written by and starring Steve Martin called "L.A. Story". In one unforgettable scene his character rushes out of his Beverly Hills mansion, jumps in his car and drives up the street one house to visit his next-door neighbor.

All of us have the constant experience of trying to get the closest parking place whenever we go to a movie, restaurant, work, etc. If we were thinking about burning calories we would take the farthest parking place. This could be an easy and frequent way to cut a few calories here and there. Every time you go to the market, movie, mall, work, you name it, park a little farther away. Make a point of taking the stairs if you are only going up one or two floors in a building.

Here's an example of how this might work to help you lose weight. If you park your car 100 yards further than you would ordinarily and walk at a leisurely pace you will burn 7.5 extra calories (on top of what you would burn lying down). Let's say that you do this at work (arriving and leaving) and at the market on the way home to pick up something to eat (arriving and leaving). That burns 30 extra calories and results in a little over 2-pound weight loss over time. How did I get this number? I divided 30 by a typical number of calories needed to maintain one pound of body weight for a sedentary individual (12). 30 divided by 12 is 2.5 or 2.5 pounds of body weight. Do you want to know how long it will take you lose this 2.5 pounds of body weight? Multiply 2.5 by 3500 and you get 8700 calories. Next you divide 8700 by 30 (calories per day) and you get 292 days. The weight will be lost faster at first and slower toward the end of the period. If you only park 100 feet further away it still burns 10 extra calories, a little under one pound lost over time.

Suppose that every time you go into a department store and need something on the second floor you make a point of taking the stairs rather than the escalator. Or if there are no stairs, then you can walk up the escalator instead of standing there and letting the escalator do all the work. At work the same thing. At home rather than asking your spouse to go upstairs to get your slippers, you walk up and get them yourself. Each time you walk upstairs you burn five calories more than if you stood while going up the escalator or elevator. Let's say that over time you average one flight of stairs per day. Doing that on a consistent basis will lose you one half-pound. The math works the same as in the previous paragraph. 5 calories divided by the 12 calories it takes to maintain one pound equals 0.42 pounds over time. I won't bore you with the "over time" calculations again. The period of time is about the same.

Table 2

Calories per hour during various activities for various weights

ACTIVITY Pounds:	120 p	140p	160p	180p	200p	220p
Sleeping, Reclining	50 cal	58	69	78	86	99
Very light: sitting	73	83	103	115	127	150
Light: walking on level, shopping, light housekeeping	143	166	200	225	250	290
Moderate: cycling, dancing, skiing, tennis	226	262	307	345	382	430
Heavy: Walking uphill, shoveling, swimming, playing basketball or football	440	512	598	670	746	840

Weigh Yourself Daily

Buy a scale. Not just any scale. It needs to be a scale with which you can't argue. My old analogue scale would move a few pounds one way or another depending upon which way I leaned. Then I would argue with it. I didn't really gain two pounds over the weekend, I'm just leaning the wrong way. You can't argue with a digital scale. A number flashes up and that's it, no argument. These can be easily obtained and are not expensive, considering what's at stake. I would suggest weighing yourself every day. This will tell you what's going on. A resistance to doing this, which many people have, is due to denial. We wish to deny that we are gaining weight, or not losing, or not doing whatever we set out to do so that we can continue eating what we want or what we have to eat. This is addictive behavior. In fact we, as we shall see later, are addicted to our food, at least to some of our foods. The subject of denial is discussed in chapter 6.

If you do weigh yourself daily your weight will fluctuate as much as 5 pounds due to the sodium content (salt) of whatever food you had that day or the day before. This is because the body requires water to dilute extra salt that we eat. One teaspoon of salt requires one quart of water to make it isotonic (the normal concentration of salts in the body fluids) and one quart of water weighs 2.2 pounds. So if you go to Uncle Harry's 80th birthday party and pig out on all those salty ordeurves, wine, and a great meal and desert and the next day you've put on 5 pounds don't worry. You may have put on a quarter of a pound but not 5.

The main reason for weighing yourself daily, or course, is the encouragement you receive when it becomes clear that what you are doing is working. The problem with weighing yourself less often, say weekly is that the saltiness of your meals can give you false information regarding the effectiveness of your program. For example, let's assume that you are doing well and losing a half-pound per week. The night before you weigh yourself you go out to your favorite Chinese restaurant and order your favorite dish that just happens to be soaked in soy sauce. Soy sauce contains large amounts of sodium, the main chemical in salt.

The next morning you weigh yourself and the scale says you've gained 4 1/2 pounds (5 pounds of salt and water minus the ½ pound you've actually lost). How discouraging. If you were weighing yourself daily you would see that weight melt away in a few days as your kidneys got rid of the extra salt and water. But you're weighing yourself every week so you don't know that you are being successful until perhaps the next week if hopefully you haven't eaten another salty meal close to your weigh-in time.

The main reason for not weighing yourself, as far as I can tell, is that you don't want to know that you're not losing weight. If you're not losing weight this is something you need to know.

I would suggest that you weigh yourself daily for ten days and then take an average of those ten weights. Add up the weights for ten days and divide by ten. If you don't want to know what the weighing shows each day, have your significant other weigh you and keep track of the weights for you.

No matter what I say here, however, some folks would rather not weigh themselves a lot. In that case the way your clothes fit will tell you everything you need to know. Jennifer whose health was at risk from her obesity had tried on many occasions to diet off her extra weight. She noticed however that as her weight was reduced she became increasingly anxious. She related her anxiety to a need for a physical barrier from people. She really could not bear to weigh herself frequently and doing so did interfere with her efforts to lose weight. I suggested that she try measuring her waist and set a certain number of inches as a goal rather than pounds. She did so and it worked for her. She was able to reduce her waist size about 10 inches without becoming anxious about it.

Cheating is mandatory

If you are going to be successful at losing weight, you are going to have to give yourself permission to cheat on your diet. Parties and celebrations are not the time to be thinking about dieting. If you are, eventually you will tire of the deprivation. Perhaps, as time passes, you may reach a point where you will be glad to give up that extra scoop of ice cream in order to further your dieting goals, but not at the beginning.

8

Calories count and the air does not contain them

What are calories? Calories are units of energy just as anything combustible is. For example a log in your wood stove of a certain size is enough energy to heat your home for a certain length of time, or a gallon of gasoline will run your car for 20 or 30 miles. A calorie is defined as enough energy to raise the temperature of one gram of water by one degree Celsius. Food is the fuel that we use to run our bodily machine and the calorie is the unit of measurement that tells us how much energy any amount of a particular food contains.

Most of us folks who fight our weight would swear that the air has calories. We seem to gain weight without eating hardly anything. Unlikely as it seems, however, the air does not have calories. Rather, we must proceed on the basis that our weight is very closely determined by the number of calories contained in the food we eat each day. Learning the caloric content of the foods that you eat will be extremely important in developing a plan to lose weight.

A good general rule to remember is that you will need 12-15 calories per pound of body weight in order to maintain your current body weight. The actual number depends on your physical activity level, the percentage of your weight that is fat, and your basal metabolism. So if you are sedentary (you sit in an office most of the day, drive to and from work, watch TV at night) use the 12 and if you are quite active (you work as a carpenter) use 15. Others will be somewhere in between.

Calories to Maintain Weight			
Weight	Active (15 cal/lb)	Still Moving (13.5 cal/lb)	Sedentary (12 cal/lb)
125	1875	1688	1500
150	2250	2025	1800
175	2625	2363	2100
200	3000	2700	2400
225	3375	3038	2700
250	3750	3375	3000
275	4125	3713	3300
300	4500	4050	3600

As an example, if you weigh 200 pounds and are sedentary you will need 200X12 or 2400 calories a day in order to maintain your weight. If you take in more that 2400 calories you will gain weight and if you take in fewer than 2400 calories you will lose weight. These numbers are very close to being correct but are not exact because they depend on many individual factors. There is a gender factor here. Women need fewer calories because their muscle mass is smaller and more of their body mass tends to be fat, which uses fewer calories than muscle. Also, your age will factor in this as the older you get the fewer calories you will need to maintain your weight.

The main point to keep in mind is that no matter how small the reduction in calories below the amount needed to maintain your weight, eventually some weight will be lost. It may take longer, but eventually you will get there. For example, suppose you are only able to reduce your caloric intake by 25 calories per day. You will lose about 2 pounds (if you are sedentary) and it will take about 8 months. 50 calories will get you 4 pounds in 8 months. 100 calories less than those needed to maintain your weight will lose you 8 pounds in about 9 months.

Calories from alcohol are a special problem

Calories from alcohol are a special problem. Alcohol is extremely caloric. A general rule is as follows: one and one half ounces of spirits (whiskey, gin, vodka), six ounces of wine, 12 ounces of beer all run around 150 calories. These are easy calories. You don't feel like you've eaten anything. Even though the body uses alcohol as a source of energy, it is not registered by the brain as food and therefore your hunger will not be satiated. Beer has a small amount of carbohydrate and protein. Wine a very small amount of carbohydrate. Liquor has nothing except alcohol unless you add a mixer, which usually doubles the caloric content of the drink. I understand that this may be a little confusing. Alcohol is a small molecule and will be absorbed into the metabolic pathways and help the body make those packets of energy discussed earlier. But it takes the larger molecules from carbohydrates, proteins, and fats to signal the brain that food is indeed on the way. I guess the point here is that the amount of calories you get from alcohol is not related to hunger. It is related to how much you drink which is related to other issues. Changing your drinking habits is a fairly easy way to cut calories with out making you hungry.

Sam is a man in his 50's being treated for depression. He had several drinks containing alcohol per day. He was not particularly concerned about his weight. He decided to stop drinking because of warnings associated with the antidepressants he was taking. Over a period of about a year he lost 53 pounds. He did not notice any change in his appetite, only that he had lost all this weight.

Donna, a 60-year-old grandmother of six, became concerned about her excessive weight, which was related to the development of arthritis is her left knee. This was interfering with her ability to play with her new granddaughter. Her Doctor recommended that she lose weight. In looking for areas in her daily food intake in which to cut down, she focused on her two drinks of spirits before dinner. First she measured the exact amount and found that she was consuming two one and one half-ounce drinks of 80 proof vodka with tonic mixer each evening. Looking up liquor in her calorie book she found that the 3 oz of 80 proof vodka accounted for 200 calories. The 8 ounces of Tonic water accounted for 80 calories. She thought that she could do without one half of one of her two drinks, and substitute diet tonic water for regular tonic water. The substitution of diet tonic water reduced the calories by 80 and the half drink reduction accounted for another 50 calories. This 130 calories maintained about 11 pounds of excess weight. She was able to accomplish this reduction in calories without noticing any change in her appetite. As she started to lose weight she was encouraged to look for other small changes that she could make in her food intake. Over a period of about one-year she was able to lose about 15 pounds. Her weight loss and some medication prescribed by her Doctor yielded a reduction in symptoms sufficient to increase her grandmotherly activities.

9

No second helpings

When I was a child and I left food on my plate, my mother used to say, "your eyes are bigger than your stomach". I contend that it was not my eyes that were bigger than my stomach, but that *her* eyes were bigger than my stomach, and she served the plates. Nevertheless we are expected to eat everything on our plates. I think that it is probably very deeply ingrained in most animals to eat up everything they can because "in nature" you never know when your next meal is coming from.

It was later in my life that, while searching for habits that would curtail my ever growing waist line, I learned that if I stuck to what I had put on my plate that I would be satisfied and I would stop gaining weight. So my eyes weren't bigger than my stomach. They knew just exactly what I needed. So I made a rule for myself. "No Second Helpings" This was difficult at first. I was husband and father of four. When we ate in restaurants I was the human garbage pail. I was expected to eat all the leftovers left by all those people whose eyes were bigger than their stomachs. And I did. After all we paid for all that food and couldn't think of letting it go to waste.

Remember the Starving Children

There is also the issue probably lurking in here that for some of us raised during and after World War II there is guilt about having too much to eat while others in the world were starving. Many of us were made to feel guilty for not emptying our plates because others in the world were starving. We were encouraged to eat more than we needed or wanted. Many of us came to realize that there eating everything on our plate could not affect world hunger, but childhood lessons continue to run deep. Of course it's always a good idea to keep in mind that others are less fortunate than we are if for no other reason than to put a check on our naturally gluttonous instincts.

In order to follow the rule of "No Second Helpings" you must serve your own plate. You should put exactly what looks to be the right amount and then that's it. No second helpings. You may be tempted to put somewhat less than the right amount but that misses the point. Put just the right amount. This is fairly easy to do at home but not when you eat out. In a restaurant you will be served whatever the owner has decided is the amount that will bring you back the next time. Unfortunately this amount is becoming larger and larger. I have found that if I ask for a take out box at the time I am served my meal that I can scrape of the extra food and make my portion "just right". If this is an embarrassing thing to do then try to become aware of that sensation of fullness that you get when your stomach is full and stop eating at that point. (You can still take the leftovers home.)

If you eat out a lot, it's going to be quite hard to lose weight, but not impossible. Once you accept the fact that each meal out is not a celebration but part of your normal routine, you can start adjusting your portions and selections of foods and start shaving calories. Chapter #11 goes into this in more detail.

Another problem that occurs on occasion is the popular potluck where everyone brings his or her favorite dish to share. One tends to want to sample everything and so we tend to serve ourselves too much. These are probably infrequent enough so that one doesn't need to worry about it.

10

Dealing with addictive foods

Coping with food addiction is different than dealing with any other addiction. This is because, of course, we can't stop eating. An alcoholic can stop drinking. Those addicted to nicotine can quit those habits, and many of us know how difficult that is. But those of us with food addictions must deal with them while we continue to eat.

I can almost guarantee that there are certain foods that you are addicted to. These are the foods that talk to you. These are the foods that call out to you while you're watching your favorite program on TV. During the next commercial you run to the fridge or the pantry and load up. Then during the next commercial you do it again. These addictive foods are different for everyone but they tend to have two ingredients in common; sugar and fat. They cannot be resisted. Mine were nuts, cookies, potato chips, chocolate of any sort, and left over birthday cakes and pies. If any of this stuff is in the house I will eat it until it's gone. Gradually I came to realize that I would not ever be able to make any impact on my weight as long as these foods were in the house. After much haggling with my wife (our children have moved on in their lives which makes it easier) we agreed that leftovers of these foods would be tossed or sent home with whoever brought them. Has anyone ever thrown a 2-pound box of Sees candy in the trash? The answer is now yes. So if your thing is ice cream, great. Have some. But don't keep a gallon of it in the freezer.

After dinner is the most difficult time for most people who struggle with their weight. This is a somewhat mysterious fact. After all we just finished a nice big nourishing meal with plenty of protein and fat and won't really feel hungry for a long time. But, we are sitting in front of the TV enjoying our evening programs and then the trips to the fridge and/or the pantry begin. The after dinner snack addiction will need attention and may be a source of significant calorie reduction.

Whatever your snacks are, they can be reduced a bit or replaced by another one lower in calories. Also, as suggested elsewhere, some oral satisfaction can be obtained with sugarless gum, toothpicks, etc. You also may wish to use a trick to end the snack time. A cup of coffee or tea, a stick of sugarless gum may be used as a signal that snack time is over.

11

Eating out

At the present time it is estimated that about 40% of all meals are eaten in restaurants. In order to compete with one another, restaurants have decided that bigger is better and that people will tend to go where they get more food for their dollar. It is therefore essential that we learn about the dietary content of restaurant food. It is also important to realize that eating in restaurants sensitizes us to ingesting large amounts of rich, good tasting food. In other words if we eat a substantial amount of rich food, then that is the only kind of food that we will desire.

In a study at Pennsylvania State University, researchers gave 51 college students four different-sized servings of macaroni and cheese-the smallest was 21/2 cups and the largest was 5 cups. The participants in the study came to the laboratory several times and were fed different serving sizes each time. They were told they could eat as much or little as they wanted. The researchers found: men ate on average 1.9 cups when served the 2 ½ cup portion, but they ate 2 ½ cups when they were served the 5 cup portion. Women ate on average 1.4 cups when served the 2 ½ cup portion, but they ate 1 ¾ when served the 5 cup portion. After the meals, participants rated their fullness the same, regardless of how much they had eaten. About half the participants didn't notice that the size of the portions were different from meal to meal. Barbara Rolls, professor of nutrition at Penn State, believes that people are being subtly driven to eat more by the size of the portions.

In another study, Lisa Young, an adjunct assistant professor in the department of nutrition and food studies at New York University weighed and analyzed servings of commonly eaten foods from restaurant chains and brand-name items in delis and compared them with recommended portion sizes recommended by the U.S.D.A. Among her findings published in the February 2002 issue of the American Journal of Public Health:

- Many restaurants served about 3 cups of pasta for an entrée, which would account for 600 calories before any sauce is added. The recommended portion size by the U.S.D.A. is 1 cup.
- A large cookie from a typical deli weighed about 4 ounces, which would account for 400-500 calories, depending on the type of cookie. A medium cookie should weigh about half an ounce, according to the U.S.D.A. That would be about 60 calories.
- A typical muffin was 6 ½ ounces but some weighed as much as 11 ounces. A medium muffin should be about 1 ½ ounces according to the U.S.D.A.
- 7-Eleven has a 64-ounce soda that contains 800 calories, an amount 10 times the size of the former small bottles of Coca-Cola.
- At Starbucks, if you want a small coffee, you have to order the "tall", which is 12 ounces. Dr. Young points out "that epitomizes what is going on in America when the tall is considered a small. They don't want to use the word small. It's taboo."

Until recently information regarding the dietary content of restaurant food was hard to come by. A book, "Restaurant Confidential", was recently published by Workman publishers written by Jacobson and Hurley of the Center for Science in the Public Interest after nine years of research into the content of restaurant food. This is a wonderful resource and should be owned by everyone struggling with his or her weight. The lists are exhaustive and include suggestions for how to make substitutions in your entrée suggestions so as to reduce caloric and saturated fat content. The results of their study are shocking, as you will see.

Caloric content of some common appetizers and snacks:

Cheese fries with ranch dressing: 3,010 calories
Fried whole onion with dipping sauce: 2,130 calories
Movie theater popcorn with butter (large): 1,640 calories
Sbarro Sausage and Pepperoni Stuffed Pizza (one slice): 880 calories
McDonalds shake (large): 1,010 calories
Burger King French fries (King size): 600 calories
Starbucks White Chocolate Mocha with whole milk (venti-20 oz): 600 calories
Cinnabon: 670 calories

Caloric content of some breakfasts:

Pancakes with syrup: 870 calories
French toast with syrup: 800 calories
Belgian waffle: 900 calories
Denny's original grand slam: 1,030 calories
Denny's farmer's slam: 1,430 calories

Caloric content of some sandwiches:

Turkey club: 740 calories
BLT: 600 calories
Reuben: 920 calories
Tuna salad: 830 calories

Caloric content of some Chinese takeout foods:

One egg roll: 190 calories
Beef with Broccoli: 1180 calories
Chicken Chow Mein: 1010 calories
Fried rice: 1,480 calories
Orange crispy beef: 1,770 calories
Sweet and sour pork: 1,610 calories
Kung pao chicken: 1620 calories

Caloric content of some Italian take-out dinners:

Fried calamari: 1,040 calories
Spaghetti with meatballs: 1160 calories
Fettuccine Alfredo: 1500 calories
Lasagna: 960 calories

Movie theater snacks

A large popcorn with butter contains 1,600 calories!
A bag of Reese's Pieces contains 1,000 calories!

These are examples of the worst caloric offenders. I present them here to bring attention to these meals with shocking amounts of calories. Many of these "snacks" contain half of a whole day's calories.

Let's see what happens if various size people, whose weights are stable, start eating one of these large snacks once a week. We will assume a sedentary life style (12 calories per pound to maintain their weight). How about a bag of Reese's pieces (1000 calories) at the Movie Theater:

150 pounds: will gain 12 pounds in about 10 months and weigh 162 pounds.
175 pounds: will gain 12 pounds in about 10 months and weigh 187 pounds
200 pounds: will gain 12 pounds in about 10 months and weigh 212 pounds

One needs to be very wary of the so-called value combinations at some of the fast food restaurants. These combos are tempting not only because of the price but because all you have to do is order a number. When you approach the counter of one of these establishments it can be very confusing and with people in line in back of you and your wife and 10 kids clamoring for their dinner what could be easier than, "I'll have six number 2s and four number 5s". The fast food chains encourage the sale of these combinations because it saves them money. This is because the labor and packaging involved in separating the portions costs more than the extra food.

At McDonalds, for example, you can order a combination of a Big Mac, Medium Fries, and a medium Classic Coke. "Not too bad", you think to yourself, "only the medium fries, and medium coke". 1250 Calories!! Hard to believe, but true. I don't mean to pick on McDonalds. All of the big chains have the same deals with a roughly equivalent caloric content.

Take the above example and order individual servings rather than the combo. Let's say a Big Mac, small fries, and a small (or any size) diet coke. 800 calories. Still shocking, but 450 calories less than the previous monstrosity. If you eat at McDonalds once a week and make this change, you will eat about 65 calories per day less. Those 65 calories maintain about 5 pounds of body weight in a sedentary individual.

Richard, a 29-year-old man with Down syndrome, is about 20 pounds overweight. His doctor is concerned about the potential for diabetes. He loves to eat at Taco Bell. He can read and write but when confronted with the huge numbers of decisions presented on the big board at the ordering counter he always opts for the number system and is proud about his ability to do it. On a recent daylong car trip the family stopped at Taco Bell for lunch. Richard, proud of his ability to independently operate in the world, marched up to the counter and ordered number 3, the Beef Gordita Combo. This included 2 beef gorditas, a taco, and a 24-ounce classic coke. This "lunch" contained 1,025 calories. Richard needs about 2,000 calories/day to maintain his current weight. Since he tends to eat three roughly equal meals per day plus a couple of snacks, he can afford to eat about 5 or 6 hundred calories at lunch. The extra 500 calories, if consumed once a week, maintains about 6 of his extra 20 pounds.

All of these restaurants, however, have meals with reasonable amounts of calories, especially if you stay away from the combo's.

Some examples:

Sandwiches:

Turkey breast with mustard, no mayo-370 calories
Roast beef with mustard, no mayo-460 calories
Chicken salad with no mayo on the bread-540 calories
Ham with mustard-560 calories

Fast foods:

Burger King chicken sandwich-550 calories, without mayo-390 calories
Burger King hamburger-320 calories, whopper Jr. 410 calories
Burger King small French fries-230 calories, medium 320 calories
Burger King biscuit with egg-390 calories

Kentucky fried chicken tender roast sandwich without sauce-270 calories, with sauce-350 calories

Kentucky Fried Chicken Triple Crunch Zinger Sandwich without sauce-390 calories
Kentucky Fried Chicken Tender Roast Sandwich with sauce and Corn on the Cob-500 calories

McDonalds Chicken McGrill without mayo 340 calories, with mayo 450 calories
McDonalds Hamburger-280 calories, Cheeseburger-330 calories
McDonalds Quarter Pounder-430 calories
McDonalds Chicken McNuggets 430 calories
McDonalds small french fries-210 calories, Medium-450 calories
McDonalds Egg McMuffin-290 calories
McDonalds Sausage McMuffin-360 calories
McDonalds Hashbrowns 130 calories

Taco Bell Chicken Fiesta Burrito-370 calories
Taco Bell Steak Fiesta Burrito-370 calories
Taco Bell Bean Burrito-370 calories
Taco Bell Chicken Chalupa Nacho Cheese-350 calories
Taco Bell Chicken Gordita Nacho Cheese-290 calories
Taco Bell Steak Gordita Baja-340 calories

Wendy's Grilled Chicken Sandwich-300 calories
Wendy's Classic Single with Everything-410 calories
Wendy's Mandarin Chicken Salad-160 calories

Mall Foods:

Starbucks Cappuccino with skim milk-110 calories
Starbucks Cafe Latte with skim milk-160 calories

Mrs. Fields: has a number of small cookies and other sweets in the 150 calorie range

Cinnebon Minibon-300 calories

Sbaro Spaghetti with Sauce-630 calories
Sbaro Cheese Pizza (one slice)-450 calories

 The point I'm trying to make here by listing these examples is that it will help a lot if you do a little research into the caloric content of what you're eating when you eat out. It will make a big difference in how many calories you conume. Also, to make the point again because it's so important, don't fall for the "value meals". They are a value for the restaurant, not for you.

12

Tricks and triggers

Most people who are habit ridden are familiar with triggers. Those situations, events, time of day, emotional events, and so on, that lead to impulses to eat, smoke, or drink. Anyone who smokes is most likely very familiar with this process. After meals is a very common time to "have to have a smoke".

Food, also, appears to have its triggers. Go to a movie theater and watch people. What are these washtub size barrels of popcorn and half gallon size sodas. It appears that going to a movie constitutes a trigger to eat popcorn, sodas, and very large boxes of candy. What happened to those little snack size boxes of milk duds they had when I was a kid? The boxes you get now would feed a small army. Many people, then, have a large dinner and then go to a movie and eat another thousand calories of junk food because of the movie trigger.

Probably the television set acts in the same way. I think many people eat while they watch TV and that the TV has become a trigger to eat for many of us.

You will need to determine what your triggers are. It will be part of your job to work on dealing with them so that they don't contribute to your weight problem. That's where tricks come in.

Tricks are what I call those methods I have developed to stop certain eating habits or to not respond to my triggers, but without feeling deprived.

There are tricks to ending the meal, hopefully before one is stuffed. I think of it as a signal that the meal is over. My signal is a cup of decaffeinated coffee. After my cup of coffee there is no more eating. I do this after every meal and after every snack. Otherwise I would want seconds and thirds.

I also use sugarless gum as a substitute for a craving food. I'm not talking about genuine hunger. If you're hungry, eat something. But if you just had a nice meal and find yourself craving more food, pop a stick of sugarless gum in your mouth. Sometimes chewing on a toothpick will take your mind off your craving.

Try tricking yourself into accepting very slight reductions in portion size. For example, try shaving half an ounce of your hamburger patty; three and a half ounces instead of four. That would save you 30 or 40 calories and you probably won't notice it.

I hesitate to even bring up the subject of pizza, which was invented by the devil to tempt us all into gluttony. Instead of tearing off piece after piece until you need to be carried away from the table, try serving yourself enough slices right away that look to be the right amount. Or if you're eating takeout at home, buy a pizza cutter and cut some slices in half. Instead of your usual four, five, or six slices, cut down by one half slice. Generally a slice of pizza will contain between about 250 and 300 calories depending on what it has on it. So if you can cut down your meal by one half slice, you will have saved about 125 to 150 calories. If you eat take out pizza once a week that half slice is maintaining 1 ½ pounds of body weight.

When serving your plate at home first serve your vegetable portion. This takes up space on your plate (and in your stomach) without using many calories. Then there isn't as much room for the more caloric entrée. Your meal may look like as much food as usual but there may be 50 or so fewer calories than previously. Remember that we're only trying to trick ourselves in to cutting out a few calories here and there in a way that we won't notice the change. Some ideas for this purpose are steamed broccoli, squash, sweet corn on the cobb without butter, green beans, Brussels sprouts, and asparagus. Frozen vegetables such as carrots, peas, green beans, corn, and mixed vegetables also serve very well for this purpose.

One trick offered by a friend who helped with this book involved his difficulty with the idea of ever giving up any of his food. He therefore devised a clever scheme. He would give up something, but only for one day. The next day he would take the treasured item back, but he would find another one to cut for one day. So far it's working and his weight is lower than it's been for years.

13

First step-stabilizing your weight

The first step in this process of losing weight is to stop gaining. This may seem like a no-brainer and not even worth going into but in my experience it is a definite step in the process and needs to be addressed as a separate issue. In fact I would take this a step further and suggest that you not even try to lose weight during this time. You are only going to stop gaining and establish what your stable weight is. This will not be easy and may take a while.

If you are gaining weight it will become clear that you are because you are weighing yourself daily and watching the numbers go up and your clothes are getting tight. You have two choices. One is to wait until you stop gaining. This presumes that you won't continually increase your food intake. The second option is to make some changes in your eating habits now to stop the gain.

By now you have familiarized yourself with the caloric content of all the foods that you tend to eat on a regular basis. You have learned how to read the dietary information on the packages of food. You have a diary in which you have kept track of what you eat and the caloric and fat content. This will allow you to make decisions regarding small changes in portions and types of foods in order to cut your daily calorie intake. Some of the following suggestions may seem like they don't accomplish much. Try to remember that every little bit adds up, perhaps to an amount large enough to stabilize your weight. These examples are only intended as tips on how to approach this issue, not what you should eat.

If you eat out a lot, try cutting out one lunch or dinner and eat at home or take your lunch with you to work that day. You may be able to cut out 4 or 5 hundred calories per week just by making such a sacrifice. Remember that 500 calories per week could be maintaining 6 extra pounds. Also, you may want to try asking for the take home box at the beginning of the meal and then you control the portion size of the meal rather than the restaurant. As mentioned previously, you probably don't want to do this if eating out is an occasional activity, but if you eat out frequently, say several times per week, then you will probably have to do something to deal with the large restaurant portion problem. Even if you don't feel comfortable asking for a box at the beginning, ask for one at the end and take a little leftover home for a snack. This will get you in the habit of asking for the box, leaving a little food but not losing it. In chapter 11 You will find more information related to eating out.

If you like fast foods, try cutting out the French fries, or split an order with a friend. These are unbelievably caloric soaked in oil as they are. Order ala Carte rather than a numbered special. This could be the fast food equivalent of serving your own plate. At least you have to make a decision regarding each portion. You could order the single patty burger or the small fries or a small diet soda (if there is such a thing).

If you just have to have that great desert that your favorite restaurant is famous for, split it with your significant other or friend.

Bread, pasta, rice, and potatoes are inherently low calorie, filling foods when combined with meats and vegetables in a balanced manner. It's what goes on them that is the problem if in large amounts. A slice of bread is about 100 calories. If you put a tablespoon of butter on it, then it becomes 200 calories. Try putting a half-tablespoon. That would cut out 50 calories. 1 ½ cups of cooked Pasta with one cup of marinara sauce is quite filling and low in calories (about 500 for a very filling meal). Pasta with cheese is quite caloric. Marie Callander's Fettuccine Alfredo for example gives you 450 calories for only a one cup meal. A medium potato contains about 100 calories. By the time we slather it with butter and sour cream it contains enough calories for a major meal all by itself. Try using somewhat less butter and sour cream. Or if you can't deal with less butter and sour cream, try half a potato. Remember every little bit helps.

Many restaurants really soak their salads in dressing. Try ordering the dressing on the side. This way you control how much fat goes on the lettuce. At home skip the salad occasionally and substitute cooked vegetables, frozen or fresh, whatever is convenient for you.

Vegetables are filling and good for you and low in calories. But if you put a rich sauce on them, they become highly caloric. Once this habit is engrained its hard to break. Rich sauces are very habit forming. Most vegetables have very pleasing flavors all by themselves. Try giving them a chance or add a little salt and pepper or other taste enhancers that won't add to the caloric content. Fruit is great for snacks, desserts, and salads. The food value is very good and the caloric content low. Many people are able to get used to the low or no fat milks. This may be another way to shave a few calories off.

Try using a sugar substitute such as Equal (NutraSweet) on your cereal in the morning. If you are in the habit of putting say 2 teaspoons of sugar on your cereal in the morning you will save a few calories.

A level-measuring teaspoon of sugar is worth 18 calories. This little substitution will save you 36 calories.

At home when you cook meat, choose the lean cut (unless you're grilling during which the fat is rendered off). You may want to trim off all the extra fat. The reduction in calories from the fattier cuts is significant. You may pay a few dollars a pound more but in the long run you will save. It's penny wise and pound-foolish to save money by eating fatty meats. Of course there are those special occasions when nothing else will do. Rather than eat deep-fried chicken, try roasting it. The fat that is mostly in the skin is rendered off but that great taste remains. You can also use the skinless legs and breasts available in most markets in recipes where you won't miss the loss of the tasty skin.

If you have, or can develop, a taste for fish, this is a low calorie complete protein with healthy fish oils (omega 3 fatty acids). There are calories to be saved compared to beef. 4 oz of ground beef (lean) contain 300 calories, 4 oz king salmon contain 200 calories, and 4 oz of halibut contain 120 calories. Suppose you substitute 4oz of halibut for 4 oz of ground beef once per week. You will save 180 calories or about 26 calories per day, enough to maintain about 2 pounds of body weight if you are a sedentary individual.

Learn to pay attention to physical cues that your body sends when you've had enough to eat—that feeling of fullness that we get in our abdomen when our stomach is full of food. Those of us who struggle with our weight tend to ignore these sensations and keep eating. If someone else has served your meal, this sensation may arrive before all the food is gone. So you must do that awful thing and waste food or if you are at a restaurant you can take the leftovers home and have them for lunch tomorrow.

14

Resting or turning eating efforts into eating habits

Once you have stabilized your weight it's time to rest. Your psyche and your body will experience this change in your eating habits as a deprivation. You need to give yourself time to get used to it. I can't give much guidance about how long. I guess the answer is when you feel comfortable with the idea of taking another step. Also when you're very confident that your weight is under control. The amount of time involved may be frustrating as you are anxious to start losing weight, but you really can't get around it. If you don't allow yourself to get used to each step in the process then you will probably sabotage the whole thing and wind up where you started or worse.

The rest period is a dangerous one for the dieter. We've accomplished our goal. We can relax for a while. Maybe we can have a little more of whatever it is that we crave. After all we can afford to eat a few extra calories since we just stopped gaining, lost several pounds, or whatever. One must be ever vigilant to maintain the new habits you have striven so mightily to obtain.

15

Making a plan to lose weight

As we've mentioned several times in earlier chapters, one pound of body weight is equivalent to 3500 calories. In other words you will have to eat 3500 extra calories to gain a pound and eat 3500 fewer calories than are required to maintain your weight to lose a pound. If you require 2400 calories to maintain your 200-pound body and you cut your intake to 2300 calories you will lose one pound in about one month (30X100 equal 3000), actually 35 days to be exact. Those 100 calories per day maintain about 8 pounds of body weight in a sedentary individual. Therefore, if you continue to consume 2300 calories rather than 2400 calories you will lose a total of 8 pounds. Remember that you are losing about one pound per month, decreasing as you go along, so this should take about one year. You will lose faster at the beginning and slower at the end. This is because at the beginning you are eating (in this case) 100 calories less than you need to maintain your weight, but as you approach your goal (8 pound loss) you are eating about what you need to maintain your new weight.

I'm sure you're thinking, "why bother?" "Why go to all that trouble to lose a measly 8 pounds and have it take a year?" That's a very good question. Actually 8 pounds is a very significant weight loss and can lead to a marked reduction is blood pressure and blood cholesterol levels. Diabetes can be helped by surprisingly small losses of weight. Also even a small loss of weight may result in a feeling of confidence with respect to further efforts toward losing more weight.

Now it's time to make a tentative decision about how much weight you want to lose. This needs to be a reasonable, reachable goal, after which you will rest again. I would suggest between 5 and 10 pounds. From the above example you can see that we're talking about 100 calories per day reduction in your daily caloric intake. This will be true no matter how much you weigh. 100 pounds or 400 pounds; if you reduce your daily caloric intake by 100 calories you will lose about 8 pounds.

Let's suppose that you've opted for the 100 calories/day and 8 pounds weight loss. Your actual amounts will of course depend upon what you decide. Now you have to find food in your daily diet that you can do without that is worth 100 calories. Sound easy? It isn't. Your body will do everything it can to keep you from eating less. So you have to kind of trick it.

The corn muffin story

I'll give an example from my own struggles. I had the habit of eating a corn muffin (left over from Sunday breakfast) soaked in maple syrup as an after dinner snack. I wasn't hungry. I just wanted that corn muffin and syrup. I calculated that the corn muffin and syrup amounted to about 300 calories. I figured that here was the place where I could get rid of a bunch of calories; wrong. No matter what I did I couldn't stop eating that corn muffin. I tried bread sticks. I'd have 2 or 3 bread sticks-150 calories, but I'd still have to have the corn muffin. Then I was having 450 calories after dinner rather than just the 300 from the corn muffin. I tried low fat popcorn. Same thing; had to have the corn muffin. I actually gained a few pounds rather than losing. I gradually had to accept that I wasn't going to be able to cut out this sweet after dinner snack I looked for a substitute. I like crunchy granola bars. One granola bar has 180 calories. If I had a granola bar I found that I didn't need the corn muffin. But to be on the safe side I threw out the extra corn muffins after Sunday breakfast. This great triumph took me about a year. After another year the corn muffins don't call out to me anymore. You're probably wondering if I lost weight. Yes, about eight pounds. I still have some to go to reach my ultimate goal and so have to find another 100 calories I can do without. Right now I'm resting. As mentioned above the rest period is dangerous. Lately I've been adding a little low fat popcorn after I have the granola bar. When I realized what I was doing and that I was in denial again, I calculated the calories. The popcorn and granola bar added up to about 300 calories. I could have been having the corn muffin. As I said before, this weight-loss business isn't easy.

It may be possible to trick your body by altering the various portion sizes. If your plate looks just as full of food but has slightly more bulk from vegetables and slightly less from meat then you may be able to shave some calories without your body rebelling.

Some people find that the low fat salad dressings work for them. I don't care for them myself preferring to use the good stuff but in smaller amounts.

So let's say that you are now taking a daily walk around the block (25 calories), have cut one ounce of wine, 2 ounces of beer, or one quarter of an ounce of spirits out of your alcohol consumption (25 calories), a small increase in vegetables and a small reduction in meat (25 calories), and once a week you don't finish your restaurant meal but bring home 175 calories of leftovers (25 calories/day). You have cut 100 calories per day and are on your way to an 8-pound weight loss.

After a time you may find that you are comfortable with these changes and wish to add to your weight loss plan. You can add: substituting halibut for ground beef once per week (26 calories/day), substitute NutraSweet for sugar on your cereal in the morning (36 calories/day), and substitute a selected menu at your favorite fast food restaurant for the combo once per week (65 calories/day). That's an additional 127 calories per day. Enough to lose about 10 additional pounds in a sedentary individual.

The above suggestions are not intended to be formulas for weight loss, only examples of how you can find areas in your own eating habits where you can make small substitutions here and there which result in calorie savings. These small savings do add up as you can see from the above. The old saw attributed to J. Paul Getty about a billion dollars here and a billion dollars there eventually adding up to real money is certainly true for calories. The small changes suggested above eventually add up to an 18-pound weight loss, which is quite significant.

If you are quite a bit overweight and wish to lose at a faster rate, I would suggest that you try losing at the slower rate first. See how it goes. You can always take away more calories later if it is comfortable to do so.

16

Resting after a weight loss

Congratulations. You've lost weight. Now the hard part starts. Keeping it off. You will probably now be tempted to use your newly acquired weight loss as a rationalization for eating more. It may go something like this: "Since I've lost all this weight it won't hurt just this once if I have another 10 pieces of pizza, three extra helpings of pie, six candy bars, etc., etc".

It is crucial now to stick to your new eating habits. This is the time to get used to your new body. Are your clothes loose? You may need to buy clothes that fit. Don't fall into the trap of saying to yourself that you'll wait until you lose some more weight before you spend all that money on new clothes. You are likely to be at this new weight for a long time before you embark on an attempt at further weight loss. Or, you may not trust that the weight will stay off, so why waste the money. Balderdash and poppycock. Buy the clothes!

This rest period is likely to last a long time. You will not be in a hurry to go through the struggles that you have just been through in the near future. The idea of finding yet more food to eat less of is not especially appealing right now. So don't. Take your time. You'll know when to start again. It's very important not to rush.

17

Holiday eating

It starts at Halloween and stops at New Years. That's two months where we give ourselves permission to overeat, especially rich foods. Most people gain considerable weight during this time. You know who you are, and how much you gain, and whether you lose it after the holidays, and how long it takes to get back to your usual weight.

Suppose you gain between three and five pounds during the holidays. You have recently embarked on a plan to lose in the neighborhood of eight pounds (or whatever your goal is) over the next year. You lose the eight pounds and then the holidays come around and you gain five back. You can see where I'm going. If you are serious about losing weight then you've got to do something about holiday eating. What that is will look different for everyone. I can only reiterate ideas already discussed. All those great food gifts people send you should be tasted and then thrown out or given away (so someone else can gain weight). Don't keep bowls of nuts and candy sitting around the house. Lighten up on the cookie making. Nothing is worse for a dieter (food challenged person) than an endless supply of cookies available during those cold December days. I'm not suggesting giving broccoli spears for Halloween treats but learn to be reasonable with yourself around holiday sweets.

I would say that the basic idea is to limit your celebratory eating to one day. Not much damage can be done in one day. It's the weeks that all of the rich candies, cookies, nuts, and cakes sit in your house and which can't be resisted that do the damage.

18

Quitting smoking

If you are planning to quit smoking, you are going to gain weight. Don't fight it. Do whatever it takes to deal with your nicotine addiction. This is by far the greatest health risk that you have. You can deal with the weight issue later after you are free of your nicotine addiction.

If you have smoked for a long time your metabolic rate has been permanently altered. You will probably reach a stable weight, which is greater than your stable weight prior to beginning smoking. Sometimes people start smoking again when they find themselves gaining, even after they have successfully quit. This is a viscous cycle. You will need to accept that your stable weight will be larger than it ever was. When you begin your weight loss efforts, you will be starting at a larger weight. But don't despair. If you're willing to plug along with some of the ideas presented here you'll get there.

19

Traveling

When we travel we suddenly regress to a very early stage in our cultural evolution. The hunter-gatherers never knew when the next meal was coming. When we are on the road we act like we don't either. A strong imperative exists which has us eat all we can at every opportunity.

A good friend and his wife recently took a one-month trip overseas. One of the options they purchased on their tour was a buffet breakfast of all you can eat. This buffet included every breakfast delicacy imaginable. My friend, who likes a big breakfast but has learned to settle for a medium size bowel of cereal with milk most mornings, found himself eating huge amounts of meats, eggs, and pastries. He reasoned that he would need the energy for all the sight seeing he would do and since this was a short period of time (a month), how much damage could he do. Well, as it turns out, a lot. About halfway through the trip he noticed that the pants he bought for the trip were getting snug. Then he noticed he was letting out his belt one notch. Then he couldn't get into the new pants at all. He started to cut down the size of his breakfast but it was too late. When he got home and resumed his pre-trip eating habits and waited a few days for his kidneys to get rid of all that extra salt, he found that he had gained four real pounds of body weight. This was very discouraging as he had been on a weight loss plan over the past two years and had managed to gradually lose 12 pounds.

We broke out the calculator and crunched the numbers. In order to gain four pounds, he had eaten 3500 times 4 equals 14,000 extra calories (on top of those needed to maintain his weight). We divided 14,000 by 28 (the number of days in the trip) and got an even 500 extra calories per day. This is not that hard to do. An extra couple of pieces of bacon, an extra scrambled egg, and an extra pastry about do it. Then we tried to figure out how long it will take to lose this weight if he simply goes back to his regular eating habits. These calculations are as follows:

In order to lose the 4 pounds he gained, he will be eating just enough calories to maintain his weight at four pounds less than his new weight. At 12 calories to maintain each extra pound he will be eating 4 times 12 equals 48 calories per day less than he needs to maintain his new weight. As can be seen from the previous paragraph, he needs a total of 14,000 calories to lose the four pounds he gained. 14,000 divided by 48 equals 292 days or roughly 10 months.

You can imagine the shock he felt. This little breakfast binge during his brief trip had not only cost him a third of the weight that he had painstakingly lost over a period of two years, but it was going to take him nearly another year to get back to where he had been.

What's that old saying? A moment on the lips, an eternity on the hips. This story is a cautionary tale about how easy it is to gain weight and how hard it is to lose it. One must be very cautious when traveling regarding this tendency to fill up at every stop.

www.ingramcontent.com/pod-product-compliance
Lightning Source LLC
LaVergne TN
LVHW041541060526
838200LV00037B/1083